# CHILDBIRTH AND PAIN RELIEF

an anesthesiologist explains your options

# CHILDBIRTH AND PAIN RELIEF

an anesthesiologist explains your options

By Sanjay Datta, M.D.

Published by:
Next Decade, Inc.
39 Old Farmstead Road
Chester, New Jersey 07930-2732 USA
www.nextdecade.com

Published by:
Next Decade, Inc.
39 Old Farmstead Road
Chester, New Jersey 07930-2732 USA
www.nextdecade.com

Cover design by Byron Design, Tucson, Arizona
Cover photograph: Byron Photography, Grand Rivers, Kentucky

© 2001 by Sanjay Datta, M.D.
Printed in the United States of America

    Library of Congress Cataloging-in-Publication Data


Datta, Sanjay.
    Childbirth and pain relief: an anesthesiologist explains your options/ by
    Sanjay, Datta.
      p.cm.
    Includes bibliographical references and index.
    ISBN 0-9626003-9-3 (pbk.)
    Anesthesia in obstetrics. 2. Analgesia. 3. Pain—Treatment. I. Title.

RG732.D277 2001
617.9'682—dc21                                      00-048985

$16.95 Softcover

# Dedication

This book is dedicated to all the mothers I was able to help during labor and delivery and also to the mothers who successfully delivered babies without my help.

# Table of Contents

# About The Author

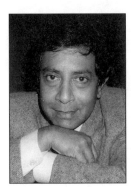 Dr. Sanjay Datta has spent the past twenty-five years as an obstetric anesthesiologist. He completed his preliminary training in England, followed by an obstetric anesthesia fellowship at McGill University in Montreal. He is currently the Director of Obstetric Anesthesia at Brigham and Women's Hospital, a Harvard Medical School affiliated hospital, a position he has held for the past eight years. His department oversees and manages the delivery of more than ten thousand babies per year, and is one of the busiest academic departments in the country. Under Dr. Datta's leadership, it is also considered one of the best in the world. In addition, Dr. Datta is currently a Full Professor in Anaesthesia at Harvard Medical School.

During his twenty-five-year medical career, Dr. Datta has also served as a Visiting Professor at many of the world's leading medical schools including the Mayo Clinic, Yale University School of Medicine, Navy Hospital in Bethesda, Columbia University, McGill University in Canada, University of Toronto, University of Basel (Switzerland), and the University of Sao Paulo (Brazil).

Dr. Datta is a member and a past President of the Society for Obstetric Anesthesia and Perinatology and a member of the

American Society of Anesthesiologists. He is also the editor/ author of over one hundred articles and numerous textbooks in the field of obstetric anesthesia.

Finally, Dr. Datta has been voted into The Best Doctors in America®, the world's preeminent physician evaluation and referral service. Best Doctors® processes more than two million evaluations through peer review surveys, and only about four percent of all U.S. doctors are included.

# Disclaimer

The purpose of this book is to provide interested individuals with a basic understanding of the complexities of childbirth and pain relief. It is presented with the understanding that the publisher and author are not engaged in rendering medical advice or other professional services in this book, and that without personal consultation the author cannot and does not render advice or judgment about a specific patient or medical condition. When medical or other expert assistance is required, the services of a competent professional should be sought.

This manual was not written to provide all the information that is available to the author/and or publisher, but to complement, amplify and supplement other texts and available information. While every effort has been made to ensure that this book is as complete and accurate as possible, there may be mistakes, either typographical or in content. Therefore, this text should be used as a general guide only, and not as the ultimate source of childbirth and pain relief information. Furthermore, this book contains current information only up to the printing date.

Information herein was obtained from various sources whose accuracy is not guaranteed. Opinions expressed and information are subject to change without notice.

The author and Next Decade, Inc. shall not be held liable, nor be responsible to any person or entity with respect to any loss or damage caused, or alleged to be caused, directly or indirectly by the information contained in this book.

If you do not wish to be bound by the above, you may return this book to the publisher for a full refund.

# Acknowledgement

During my twenty-five years of obstetric anesthesia service I have had the pleasure of meeting many wonderful expectant mothers, nurses, obstetricians along with my colleagues, including residents and faculty members. Their encouragement planted the seed for the germination of this book. I will always be thankful to my mentor, Dr. Phillip Bromage, who encouraged me to be an obstetric anesthesiologist. My wife Gouri and daughter Nandini's continuous support has been vital. Finally, I would like to thank Mrs. Elizabeth Kiernan, who was instrumental in helping me put this manuscript together. Thank you for keeping me cool and calm.

# Preface

My twenty-five years of experience as an obstetric anesthesiologist began in the famous Boston Lying-In Hospital, the first maternity hospital in the world to use ether anesthesia for pain relief during childbirth. This hospital has seen the days of "Twilight Sleep" and natural childbirth using techniques pioneered by Grantly Dick-Read and Fernand Lamaze, and later made spinal anesthesia and epidural analgesia and anesthesia popular for relief of labor and delivery pain. In 1981 I moved to the Brigham and Women's Hospital (BWH), next to the Boston Lying-In Hospital, where I was promoted to the head of obstetric anesthesia. Also at that time, Harvard Medical School helped me fulfill a lifelong ambition by rewarding me the highest-ranking title in academic medicine, Professor of Anaesthesia. This position has introduced me to many expectant mothers who have good questions and very valid concerns regarding anesthesia and pain relief used during delivery.

I have written this book to help you, the expectant mother, sort through the different anesthetic (intense sensory and motor block) and analgesic (less intense sensory block with minimal motor block) options that are available today. To help you do so; I describe the methods for providing pain relief during labor and delivery and identify the advantages and disadvantages of each method. I also discuss techniques for cesarean deliveries and considerations for situations such as systemic disease, back problems, and cervical incompetence. I hope that by reading this book you will be better equipped to choose anesthesia and analgesia methods that are right for you; however, I also encourage you to attend childbirth classes and ask your instructor any other questions you may have.

Sanjay Datta, M.D., FFARCS (Eng)

# Introduction

So, you are expecting a baby! If this is your first baby, you will need help learning about your pain relief options for both vaginal and cesarean (abdominal) deliveries. In this book, we will explore the following pain relief options for labor and delivery:

- Controlled breathing and focus, used in place of anesthesia and pain-relief medicines in natural childbirth;

- Pain-relief medicines, injected into veins or muscles;

- Regional anesthesia and analgesia techniques, including continuous spinal, epidural, and combined spinal epidural (also known as a walking epidural); and

- General anesthesia.

Choosing a birthing method, and its associated pain relief options, is a personal decision. As an expectant mother, you should consider the advantages and disadvantages of all methods to help you decide which method is best for you. Whichever method you choose, be sure to deliver your baby under the guidance of an experienced midwife or obstetrician.

# Pain During Childbirth: Dispelling the Myths

For a long time, women delivered babies without any options for relieving pain. The agony of pain and delivery has always been regarded in the Old Testament as the outcome of the primal curse pronounced by God upon Eve after the fall. "Unto the woman," God said in Genesis 3,16, "I will greatly multiply thy sorrow and thy conception; in sorrow thou shalt bring forth children." In the Old Testament, there are several references to this heritage of pain—for example, in Isaiah 26,17: "Like as a woman with child, that draweth near the time of her delivery, is in pain and crieth out in her pangs."

For centuries, the childbirth process has been associated with gods, ghosts, evil spirits, and taboos. Many unusual labor and

delivery practices developed, including the use of parts of cas-
sowary birds and swamp eels to make the birth canal slippery.
Magic, superstitions, and voodoo also had their place in childbirth among the old cultures.

Over the years, people began questioning the role of pain in
childbirth. The discovery and acceptance of painless labor had a
slow beginning, however. For example, in 1591, a pregnant
woman named Euphaine Macalyane helplessly asked her midwife
for a remedy to allay the pangs of her labor. James VI, the ruler
of Scotland at that time, ruled Euphaine Macalyne's request a sin
and the gentle lady was burned alive on a public pier to make a
point to other women who might try to evade the curse of Eve.

Fortunately for expectant mothers today, pain relief during
labor and delivery is an accepted and expected part of the childbirth process. This sentiment is embraced by the American
College of Obstetrics and Gynecology, in their committee opinion #118: "Labor results in severe pain for many women. There
is no other circumstance where it is considered acceptable for a
person to experience severe pain, amenable to safe intervention,
while under a physician's care. Maternal request is a sufficient jus-
tification for pain relief during labor."

# Physiological Changes During Pregnancy

**B**efore we look at the options for pain relief during labor and delivery, let's first explore some of the changes that happen in the body during pregnancy. Expectant mothers go through remarkable physical and emotional changes that become more pronounced as the pregnancy progresses. Some of these changes are so significant that a renowned British obstetric anesthesiologist, Dr. Selwyn Crawford, referred to the pregnant woman as the "third sex." In this section, I will briefly describe only those changes that significantly relate to anesthetic techniques and medications.

# Heart and Circulation

Because the expectant mother shares some part of her blood with her fetus, her cardiovascular system goes through remarkable changes. Her plasma volume is increased by 50%, whereas her red blood cells increase by only 18%. This situation—sometimes referred to as "anemia in pregnancy"—involves a simple dilution of the total number of red blood cells; when bleeding occurs, less red blood cells will be lost per milliliter of blood. This acts as a safety net to accommodate a moderate amount of blood loss during vaginal and abdominal (cesarean section) deliveries.

Various chemicals increase during pregnancy, causing the blood vessels to dilate and blood to circulate more easily throughout the fetus. Despite the increased blood flow, blood pressure does not change significantly. The heart has to work very hard to handle the enormous increase in blood volume. The heart works it's hardest about 24–28 weeks into the pregnancy, peaking just after delivery.

Blood also coagulates more readily during pregnancy. Some women experience pain in their legs; this pain may be a sign of blood clotting. Early diagnosis and treatment of this condition will prevent embolism.

The enlarged uterus compresses the two large blood vessels in front of the backbone, causing some expectant mothers to feel light-headed and sweaty; some lose consciousness. If the expectant mother lies on her back, her blood pressure will drop, which alleviates the lightheadedness; however, a decrease in blood pressure also means a decreased flow of blood to the baby. To minimize the drop in blood pressure, pregnant women are encouraged to sleep on their sides and, during labor, should lie on their sides after receiving regional analgesia, regional anesthesia, or general anesthesia.

The increased blood volume and dilation of the blood vessels also cause the face, throat, vocal cords, and leg and arm veins to swell. The gums and nasal passages will also swell and bleed easily. For mothers who need assistance breathing during labor or delivery (for example, during emergency cesarean deliveries under general anesthesia), anesthesiologists use small breathing tubes and try to avoid excessive manipulation of the nose while inserting the tubes.

## Respiratory System

Respiratory system changes include an increase in the breathing rate; expectant mothers may sometimes feel a shortness of breath, especially during exertion. The growing uterus pushes the diaphragm up and the lungs expand forward; however, the total lung capacity remains the same. For these reasons, regional anesthesia and analgesia techniques, where the mother remains awake and is able to control her breathing, are recommended over general anesthesia, where the mother is unconscious.

## Stomach and Bowels

Although physicians differ in opinion regarding changes to the stomach and bowels, most believe that when pain-killing medications are given to women for labor and delivery pain, stomach movement decreases, thereby increasing the fluid and food content in the stomach. During a routine ultrasound performed on a woman in labor, chunks of solid food were found even though the woman hadn't eaten in almost two days.

A full stomach during labor and delivery can be a significant problem if an emergency cesarean delivery needs to be performed and general anesthesia is administered. In this case, a breathing tube must be inserted down the mother's trachea. Large food particles may interfere with the insertion of the breathing tube, endangering both mother and baby. Stomach content can travel through the esophagus to the trachea; inhaled stomach content can cause damage to the lungs. As a precaution before administering any anesthesia—regional or general—we routinely give a drug intravenously and antacid by mouth to help decrease the stomach content and acidity.

## Sensitivity to Anesthesia

Pregnancy hormones, especially progesterone, may cause expectant mothers to be more sensitive to both local and general anesthetics. Knowing this, anesthesiologists adjust the doses of general and local anesthetic medications accordingly.

## Musculoskeletal Systems

The hormone relaxin is responsible for relaxing ligaments and for softening collagenous tissues such as cartilage and connective tissue. These changes might explain the increased incidences of back pain during pregnancy and the postpartum period.

## Eyes

For some women, the corneas may swell, interfering with the wearing of contact lenses. Lenses should be removed during labor and delivery.

## Emotions

Psychological effects of pregnancy vary greatly from woman to woman. There is no doubt that there are significant changes in sex hormones during pregnancy, as gestation progresses and immediately after delivery. Some women experience apprehension, anxiety, and fear during pregnancy. Stress hormones can affect the pain perception of the expectant mother; anesthesiologists monitor these changes closely and adjust the anesthesia techniques accordingly.

## Are These Changes Permanent?

You'll be happy to know that the physical changes described above are not permanent. The circulatory, musculoskeletal, and respiratory systems, as well as the stomach and bowels, gland functions, and eyes, return to normal a few days to a few weeks after the delivery of the baby.

# Natural Childbirth

Natural childbirth is the delivery of a baby using concentration and breathing techniques to control pain rather than relying on the assistance of medications. Two people that were instrumental in introducing natural childbirth to the modern world are Grantly Dick-Read and Fernand Lamaze.

## Erasing the Fear: Grantly Dick-Read

Grantly Dick-Read was famous for his book, *Childbirth Without Fear.* He believed that if childbirth was natural and was not associated with fear and tension, women could look forward to their deliveries with anticipation rather than apprehension.

Dick-Read completed his residency training in England's

White Chapel Hospital in the early 1900's. One day, he was called by an expectant mother in labor. He describes his first observations upon arriving at the woman's home as follows: "My patient lay covered only with sacks and an old black skirt. The room was lit by one candlestick in the top of a beer bottle on the mantle shelf. In due course, the baby was born. There was no fuss or noise. Everything seemed to have been carried out according to an ordered plan. There was only one dissension; I tried to persuade my patient to let me put the mask over her face and give her some chloroform when the head appeared and dilation of the outlet was obvious. She, however, resented the suggestion and firmly but kindly refused to take my help. It was the first time in my short experience that I had ever been refused when offering chloroform. As I looked at her, I saw an expression on her face that showed she hoped she hadn't hurt my feelings by refusing the offer. As I was about to leave some time later, I asked her why she would not use the mask. Then, shyly, she turned to me and said, 'It didn't hurt. It was meant to, wasn't it, doctor?'" This simple question had a tremendous impact on Dick-Read and led to a turning point in his career. From then on, he vowed to dispel the myth that pain was a necessary companion to childbirth.

In relation to birth without pain, one of the matrons from Maternity Hospital in London told him, "The more I see of this natural childbirth, the more I am persuaded that education is what really matters. The outstanding difference with your technique is that women seem to know their job before they start. They understand why relaxation helps and why it prevents pain in labor." This scenario could be observed from the corridor of the maternity floor—yelling was heard from some rooms, whereas in other rooms the patients belonging to Dick-Read were quiet and peaceful. Dick-Read visited America in 1946 to share his philosophy, where it was enthusiastically embraced.

## Four Emotional States of Labor

Dick-Read suggested that there are four emotional states that mother's experience during labor and delivery: elation, relaxation, inattentiveness, and exaltation. He believed every one of these states has its purpose and that proper support is necessary throughout the process to control both sensory and motor impulses for a painless delivery.

### *Elation*

Elation is associated with the onset of labor. According to Dick-Read, the onset of real labor is marked by the beginning of short, rhythmical contractions. If the expectant mother is well prepared for labor and stays relaxed, she should not feel any pain. His advice was, "Fears and other emotional stresses are the great enemies of childbirth. Even women who are well prepared and unafraid may be placed under a great deal of emotional stress by uncooperative surroundings or staff and unnecessary interventions. Neither say, do, nor insinuate anything that will stimulate anxiety or fear." Dick-Read believed that partners or other attending staff were good supportive people at this stage.

## *Relaxation*

As labor progressed, Dick-Read encouraged mothers to relax. He believed that the proper relaxation of upper and lower parts of the body—and, most importantly, the mind—became the hallmark of pain relief during the first stage of labor. He taught expectant mothers that they could help relax their bodies and minds and minimize or control the pain of contractions by taking deep breaths when uterine contractions first begin. He also felt that quiet surroundings were a very important factor in the success of this method.

Toward the end of the first stage, close to delivery, physical tension may manifest itself as back pain. This back pain may increase the fear of labor. Dick-Read found that deep, slow breathing exercises at this time helped relax the laboring mothers.

## *Inattentiveness*

Inattentiveness is the classical picture of the second physical stage of labor, the delivery of the baby. During this stage, the mother, as Dick-Read describes, "demonstrates the relative inactivity of her senses of discretion and discrimination; she becomes oblivious to her surroundings and careless of her appearance, expression, and speech. Normally—that is, in the absence of any dominating fear—she is devoid of any consciousness of herself and employs all her energies in the fulfillment of the immediate purpose." Dick-Read observed several common emotional statements uttered by expectant mothers very close to delivery, including "I have had enough," "I am completely exhausted and cannot possibly go on," and "Will you please help me."

At the very end of the second physical stage of labor, crowning occurs. At this point, mothers typically experience a burning sensation in the perineum. Dick-Read felt that tremendous encouragement and support were necessary from the attendants to divert this frightening feeling. Dick-Read beautifully described a mother's experience during this stage:

> "Eight years previously, at eight months pregnancy, she delivered twins by forceps. One had died and the remaining twin was brain damaged. She had come under my care for this birth, and was very nervous and alarmed about it all. But her labor went well, and there was not much discomfort until near the end of the first stage. Then she began to feel a certain amount of discomfort low down in the back, which was different from any previous sensation. Then the really interesting part of her labor began. She had a prolonged and good contraction, lost her smile, and became a serious woman starting her second stage. She flung her head back, and when I looked to see whether there was any change at all down below, she said 'Oh take off those clothes—it is quite impossible to be a lady now!' She lost all her natural reserve and shyness and the rather unusual refinement of speech that

characterized her. She had one or two more similar contractions, and I said, 'Now, I want you to draw a deep breath and find out whether you have any inclination to bear down.' She tried this and found that it was only pleasant. From that moment onward, I saw one of the most perfect examples of what I have so frequently described as the inattentiveness of the second stage. Her natural, quiet voice and controlled self disappeared, and she seemed to alter in every way. She paid no attention whatever to the dishevelment of her hair, the position of her clothes, the position of herself. Her eyes were half closed; between the contractions she passed into a quiet, sleepy condition, not answering when spoken to. After a time she had vent to an exaggerated groan, because it was nature's demand that she not relax the tension too quickly. 'It isn't a question of pain; it is this frightful feeling I am going to burst down below,' she said. I assured her that she was not going to burst down below, and her reply was, 'You don't know.' She generally became aggressive; a different woman altogether, but still assured me that it was not a question of pain. I added, 'Are you quite sure you are having no pain?' She looked wildly at me again, grasped my arm, and said, 'Pain? What do you call pain? The whole damn thing is painful—you ought to know it by now.' I asked her why she has not taken her gas, then. She said, 'Oh, it isn't really pain. Let's get the thing over—I am sick of it. Can't you do something?' That was her sort of behavior the whole way through. She was certainly not a woman who was conscious of what she was doing entirely, and certainly not the Mrs. X I had known for five or six years as a rather mild, gentle, and refined person in her manner. Here was the changed woman whose consciousness had been driven below the normal level, whose powers of discretion and discrimination were dulled and whose sensory receptors were inhibited. When the baby arrived, it was quite an astonishing picture. Mrs. X came out of that inattentive state, and I said, 'Here is your little girl.' In a flash, her restrain disappeared and she was wreathed in the smile of incomprehensible happiness."

### Exaltation

Exaltation is associated with the third physical stage of labor, the delivery of the placenta. The woman Dick-Read previously described had completely changed her emotion and behavior after seeing her baby. Her happiness and the expression of delight were so dramatic that the birth of the child, which marks the transition from the second physical stage of labor to the third stage, is associated with a state of exaltation.

In natural childbirth, a few women noted that the delivery of the afterbirth was an uncomfortable and painful process.

## Relaxation Techniques—
## Effective but Time Consuming

Grantly Dick-Read's personalized, hands-on relaxation technique was very effective, but time consuming to teach and learn. It became apparent to doctors that if they taught each mother personally and accompanied her through the entire delivery process, they could accommodate very few expectant mothers in their practice. For example, Dr. Harlon F. Ellis, an ardent supporter of Dick-Read's, taught the technique between 1958 and 1968 to expectant mothers at the Los Angeles County Hospital, one of the largest obstetric hospitals of the time. In 1968, he moved out of the Los Angeles area; his natural childbirth practice had grown so large he thought living in a less populated area would provide more time for his own family.

Dick-Read acknowledged that the pain these women experienced during this stage was real, and referred to the delivery of the placenta as a miniature labor. He stressed that proper support for the expectant mother was also very important at this stage.

# Preparing the Mind: Fernand Lamaze and the Pioneers of Psychoprophylaxis

Psychoprophylaxis, the preparation of the mind to deal with pain naturally, has and is still being used for pain relief during labor and delivery.

## Psychoprophylaxis–Roots in Hypnotism?

One of the pioneers of psychoprophylaxis was French physician Dr. Jean Martin Charcot, who was well known in the nineteenth century for his work on hypnotism and hysteria. Dr. Charcot pointed out that a state of intensity could be obtained to allow surgeries to be performed and to alleviate pain during labor. Together with fellow physician Dr. Bernheim, Dr. Charcot lifted the status of hypnosis from its magical stage to charlatanry.

Physicians during this period believed that hypnosis was safe for the mother and the baby and that its use resulted in a shorter labor. However, hypnosis had a few drawbacks—it was not successful in every case and experts were not readily available, especially good ones with documented success.

Other early psychoprophylaxis techniques included mesmerism, sometimes known as "magnetic sleep." In the mid-1800's, Dr. J. P. Lynell at the Manchester Lying-In Hospital brought an expectant mother to the hospital a week before her labor began and induced a mesmeric sleep for pain relief, in anticipation for a pleasant sleep during labor. On her delivery day, she was kept in a sleepwalking state and was brought back to a wakeful state at the moment of delivery. She delivered without pain, then was mesmerized back for a comfortable rest. This method met with great resistance—other physicians called this practice a great folly; the general public objected so strongly to this method that they condemned the editor of a journal in which an article promoting the method was published.

Amid drawbacks and objections, hypnosis and "magnetic sleep" gradually gave way to psychoprophylaxis, as we know it today, the positive suggestion technique.

Dr. Paul Joire of Lille, France declared in 1899 that "pain is not an essential feature of delivery and serves no useful physiological function. In fact, it is not uncommon for contractions to start long before pain, and the first stage of labor is characterized by such painless contractions." He further explained that positive suggestions may help alleviate labor pain, and supported this belief by describing women who could feel the lips of their vaginas draw apart as their babies' heads were delivered, but felt no pain. The famous Ivan Pavlov from Russia, who in 1920 investigated the physiological explanations of hypnosis and positive suggestions, further supported Dr. Joire's theory.

## Fernand Lamaze: Father of Psychoprophylaxis

Fernand Lamaze documents his work with psychoprophylaxis in his book, *Painless Childbirth: The Lamaze Method.* This book was translated by Dr. L. R. Celestin and was published in the United

States in 1970. In this book, a woman describes her childbirth experience with the Lamaze method as follows: "I gave birth to Thomas by the psychoprophylaxis method called childbirth without pain. When friends say to me, 'Well, did you feel nothing?' I reply, 'Quite the opposite, I felt everything, and that is the wonderful part of it…the amazing experience in which each second has remained imprinted in my memory and in which pain has simply found no place.'"

Lamaze believed that to prevent pain during childbirth, expectant mothers must be prepared for this process. The mind must be trained so that uterine contractions can be perceived as a series of understood processes rather than simple pain. The teaching should be practical and relatively easy to use in the hospital during labor.

The Lamaze method concentrates on removing any detrimental focus and limiting the spread and duration of pain. For this method to be successful, Lamaze believed he must first help women understand the labor process and then help them form new conditioned reflexes by teaching them a new way to breathe during labor. Dr. Lamaze described the importance of the breathing exercises—a series of quick, shallow breaths—as follows: "Normal respiration works by an inborn reflex. By modifying the rhythm of breathing, a conditioned reflex is initiated as a sort of 'branch' of the normal reflex. The repeated teaching of this new respiratory style leads to the formation of a new conditioned reflex, which we may call the contraction-respiration reflex." Dr.

Lamaze used uterine contractions as an analgesic maneuver to divert attention from the pain; the contractions become a signal for a specific type of breathing, and no more remain the center of pain.

In today's Lamaze childbirth preparation classes, between 6 and 12 expectant mothers and their partners gather for 12–16 hours, spread over a few weekly sessions, to learn the Lamaze technique. In addition to breathing exercises, Lamaze certified instructors teach relaxation, focus, and massage techniques to ease pain, describe the labor and birth process, and provide information about breastfeeding, healthy lifestyles, and medical procedures such as epidurals and other anesthesia choices. Because of their well-rounded content, Lamaze classes are helpful for any expectant mother, whether she plans to deliver her baby naturally or with the help of pain relief medications or anesthesia. For more information on finding a local Lamaze class, you can check with your hospital or birthing center or contact Lamaze International.

## Giving Birth in Water

Another natural childbirth option that has recently become more popular is the water birth. Water births provide a calm, relaxing atmosphere for both the expectant mother and her newborn.

## What is a Water Birth?

Water births are based on a belief that humans have a natural alliance with water, and that babies who are born in water recuperate faster from the stress of birth.

In a water birth, the expectant mother sits in a pool of warm water in a quiet, dimly lit room. Soothing music plays in the background to help calm her. The practitioner calmly talks her through the birth; when the baby emerges, the practitioner gently hands the baby to the mother.

Barbara Harper, an author and practitioner of water births, believes there is a direct connection between human beings and aquatic mammals that makes water birthing a natural choice. She describes this relationship in her book, *Gentle Birth Choices*, as follows: "Human beings are composed primarily of water, and many special characteristics we have link us to aquatic mammals; perhaps we carry the memory of a time when the human species had an 'aquatic interlude'... Human beings' natural alliance with water is best witnessed by observing babies who can swim naturally and easily before they learn to sit up or crawl."

## When Did Water Birthing Originate?

The history of water birthing goes back as far as Aristotle, who observed the importance of water in life. Many cultures throughout history have shared an awareness of water and its role in the birthing process. Ancient Egyptians believed that people who were born in the water became priests and priestesses. Ancient Minoan art depicts the special relationship between dolphins and humans; Minoans believed that dolphins stayed close to expectant mothers until they delivered. Women in Indian tribes all over the world gave birth in tidal pools and shallows along oceans and rivers. Today, couples in Russia travel to the coast of the Black Sea to deliver their babies; there, they learn yoga and healthy living and they deliver their babies in the sea with dolphins swimming nearby.

## Is Water Birthing for You?

Ms. Harper describes water births as uncomplicated and fulfilling experiences. She feels that babies who are born in the water have more time to relax and recuperate from the stress of birth than babies who are born in more conventional settings, such as hospital delivery rooms. Many women consider water births to be more comfortable and calming than other delivery methods, and frequently reported experiencing less pain.

Other people, such as Dr. Robbie E. David Floyd, feel that water birthing is not for everyone. In the foreword of Barbara Harper's book, Dr. Floyd remarked, "It is true that many women will not want the choices this book offers. The epidural rate stands at 80 percent, not because doctors everywhere are forcing epidurals on unwilling victims but because the majority of birthing women ask for, and often insist upon, the mind-body separation the epidural creates."

There are several reasons for the popularity of the epidural analgesia and other anesthesia and pain relief techniques used during labor and delivery, as we will explore soon. I will reiterate that choosing a birthing method is a personal decision, one that I hope this book will help you make. In the next chapter, I will focus on what is considered a more conventional delivery method—that which takes place in a hospital, using some combination of anesthesia and pain-relief medication.

# Births Assisted by Anesthesia and Pain Medication

Whether this is your first child or your fifth, you may feel that natural childbirth is not for you. If you have tried natural childbirth before and you could not make it through delivery without the help of a pain-killing medicine, do not think you have failed. Dr. Ronald Melzack, a psychologist who studied the pain phenomenon among pregnant women, found that mothers who received prepared childbirth training had lower pain scores on the McGill University pain scale than those who had received no such training. However, the effects of prepared childbirth training were relatively small and most women requested epidural analgesia anyway.

In many hospital delivery rooms, natural childbirth is passé. Twenty-five years ago, some women felt inadequate if they asked for pain medication while giving birth. The modern mother-to-be feels differently; she finds no shame in demanding drugs in pursuit of a less painful delivery. "I am not a hero," explains one woman who recently gave birth to her first child. "It seems silly to me to encourage someone to go through pain that isn't necessary."

Childbirth that takes place in a hospital setting is typically accompanied by pain relief medication given by midwives, nurses, or obstetricians, or analgesia and anesthesia administered by anesthesiologists.

## How Did Drug-Assisted Births Begin?

It is unknown who started using pain relief medication for labor and delivery, although myths and old stories give us clues. We do know that opium and Indian hemp were used in Egypt and throughout the East for pain relief as far back as 5000 years ago. Marco Polo and other sailors from Europe raved about India and its fertile opium farms. Merchants came to India by ship and camel to bring this merchandise back home to Europe.

Greeks used to mix opium with wine to ease the pain of surgery. It has been inferred that the Wise Men brought myrrh to the infant Jesus not only as a gift for the Son of God but to ease the labor pains of the Virgin Mary. Fredrich Wilhem Serturner, from Germany, was the first person to derive morphine from the opium plant. He named morphine after the god of dreams, Morpheus.

## Anesthesia's Early Use During Surgery

In the late 1880's, a psychiatry resident named Sigmund Freud was very interested in the cocaine that was brought to Austria by members of an expedition from the eastern slopes of the Andes, Peru, and Bolivia. Freud learned that Peruvian surgeons knew the local anesthetic properties of cocaine for a long time; they often chewed the coca leaves with lime during surgery, then spit on the site of the surgery to numb the wound. Dr. Freud suggested his colleague Dr. Karl Koller try this drug as an anesthetic during eye surgery.

Intrigued after reading Freud's published works on cocaine's anesthetic properties, Dr. Koller swallowed some cocaine himself and immediately experienced its powerful effect on his lips and tongue. By the 1890's, he was using cocaine in eye drops during eye surgeries at Mount Sinai Hospital in New York City. Dr. Freud's and Dr. Koller's early work led to cocaine's ultimate use as a spinal anesthetic during general surgery and childbirth.

# How Do Anesthesiologists Prepare for Participating in Childbirth?

Obstetric anesthesiologists have a significant responsibility— to relieve pain during and after labor and vaginal deliveries or cesarean births. To prepare for this responsibility, anesthesiologists undergo thorough training at recognized medical schools (like any other medical doctor), followed by an internship and three years of anesthesia residency approved by the American Board of Anesthesiology. Some of them will spend one more year of training in a subspecialty, as a fellow (fourth-year resident). At Brigham and Women's Hospital, an obstetric anesthesia fellowship is very popular; it is a joint fellowship program with Massachusetts General Hospital and takes one-year to complete. This fellowship program prepares obstetric anesthesiologists to care for high-risk mothers and newborns in a tertiary care center (an intensive care unit).

# When Will You Meet the Anesthesiologist?

Anesthesiologists typically meet the expectant mothers after they have been admitted to the hospital. If you are suffering from systemic diseases or back problems with Harrington rods (used to treat scoliosis), you should see an anesthesiologist long before you go into labor. The anesthesiologist will take your medical

# What is Cervical Incompetence?

Cervical incompetence is one of the causes of pre-term deliveries and also midterm miscarriages. The expectant mother's cervix has either dilated prematurely, or is too thin (effaced). In either case, cervical cerclage is done to prevent pre-term labor and miscarriages. This procedure involves stitching (suturing) the cervix, and is usually done when expectant mothers are 12–14 weeks pregnant. Both regional and general anesthesia can be used for this procedure. At Brigham and Women's Hospital, spinal anesthesia is the preferred method for this surgery. The women are conscious, thereby greatly diminishing the likelihood of nausea, vomiting, and aspiration of stomach content.

In routine cases, the sutures are removed 37–38 weeks into the pregnancy, usually with no need for anesthesia. However, in rare cases analgesics and tranquilizers may be necessary. Occasionally, spinal or general anesthesia is used.

history, ask you some questions, and help you choose an anesthesia or pain relief option that is right for you. If necessary, the anesthesiologist will also include your obstetrician in this decision. In addition to labor and vaginal deliveries and cesarean deliveries, anesthesiologists are also involved when a cervical cerclage procedure is performed for cervical incompetence.

# Stages of Labor

The first stage of labor is characterized by the following events:

1. Contractions occur at very regular intervals.

2. The cervix dilates.

3. Intervals between contractions gradually shorten.

4. The intensity of each contraction gradually increases.

5. There is increased discomfort and pain in the abdomen and back.

Unless circumstances advise otherwise, the obstetric team will perform a vaginal examination at this stage to:

• Determine whether the amniotic membrane surrounding the baby is intact.

• Measure the softness and extent of cervical dilation, in centimeters.

• Determine which part of the baby is closest to the birth canal.

• Determine how far the baby has come through the birth canal.

• Examine the mother's pelvic structure to determine how long the mother will be in labor.

- Examine the expansion of the vagina and the firmness of the perineum to determine when it is appropriate to begin pushing.

The first stage of labor lasts from the initial regular contractions associated with cervical dilation to a fully dilated (10 centimeters) cervix. Controversy exists among obstetricians about the timing of an epidural analgesia. I prefer making epidural analgesia available whenever an expectant mother desires pain relief, as long as her obstetrician or midwife is comfortable with the plan.

The second stage of labor begins with a fully dilated cervix and ends with the delivery of the baby. The third stage consists of the delivery of the placenta.

# Pain-relief Medicines, Yesterday and Today

Today, pain relievers, including those derived from opium or other synthetic drugs, are administered in one of the following ways:

- Subcutaneously, where the drug is injected just beneath the skin. Subcutaneous pain relievers are not widely used because of their ineffectiveness.

- Intramuscularly, where the drug is injected into a muscle. Intramuscular pain relievers are not used as often as intravenous pain relievers are because they do not work as quickly.

- Intravenously, where the drug is injected into a vein. Intravenous pain relievers are fast acting and can be given as a continuous intravenous infusion, where the drug is continuously dispensed in steady, measurable amounts through an intravenous tube, or through patient-controlled intravenous analgesia, where the expectant mother releases small amounts as she needs them by pushing a button.

Let's explore some of the pain relievers, tranquilizers, local anesthetics, and other medications used during labor and delivery. In the following list, drug brand names (names known in the marketplace) are listed first, followed by their generic names (names given to families of drugs), where appropriate.

## Pain Relievers

### Morphine

Morphine became a popular drug for labor and delivery pain relief beginning in the early 1900's. Morphine was often combined with scopolamine to invoke what was called "Twilight Sleep," a popular technique used in the Boston Lying-In Hospital until 1973. This technique combined the benefits of morphine (as a pain reliever) and scopolamine (called "the amnesia drug").

## Taking Charge: Patient-Controlled Intravenous Analgesia

Patient-controlled intravenous analgesia, or medication the expectant mother administers to herself whenever she feels she needs relief, is becoming widely accepted. With this technique, a needle is placed into a vein in the arm, along with a soft plastic catheter. The needle is removed and the plastic catheter stays behind. The expectant mother controls the amount of medication she receives by pushing a button attached to the intravenous tube.

When women are empowered to dispense their own medication, they typically use much less than is used in the continuous infusion, which in turn reduces the amount of medication that is transferred to the baby.

Because of the powerful amnesic effect of scopolamine, the expectant mothers did not remember even significant amounts of pain during labor.

The major disadvantage of Twilight Sleep was related to the drug scopolamine, which was associated with several side effects: loss of initiative, the feeling of helplessness, suppression of all inhibitions, visual and auditory hallucinations, marked excitement, and delirium. In between contractions, the expectant mothers would sleep; however, during contractions some of them would thrash around so much that they had to be restrained.

When I first came to the Boston Lying-In Hospital, I was amazed to see women with their hands and feet tied to their beds, especially considering I had just come from Royal Victoria Hospital in Montreal, a place where epidural analgesia was already popular. Because of these side effects, the popularity of scopolamine dwindled, along with the "Twilight Sleep" technique.

Compared to other drugs that are destroyed by the body in a short time, morphine lingers in both the mother's and the baby's blood for a long time. In high doses, the drug can cause respiratory depression in the babies and is therefore no longer used in many hospitals.

### Barbiturates

Combinations of morphine and barbiturates were very popular in the past for pain relief; however, barbiturates are no longer used because they can impair the sucking reflex of the baby.

### Demerol (Meperidine)

Demerol (meperidine) was, at one point, the most widely used labor and delivery analgesia. Despite this drug's effectiveness as a pain reliever, it is becoming less popular because of its possible negative effects on the baby. If this drug is administered too close to delivery, or if too large a dose is given, this drug can cross the placenta and may cause respiratory and motor depression in the baby and lower Apgar scores.

# Apgar Scores— What Do They Mean?

While anesthesia techniques were undergoing revolutionary changes, the mother of obstetric anesthesia, Virginia Apgar, arrived on the scene. Dr. Apgar developed what is called the Apgar score, which is used all over the world to evaluate babies one minute after delivery and again five minutes after delivery.

A baby is observed in five areas: appearance, pulse, facial expression (grimace), activity level, and respiration. A score from 0 to 2 is assigned for each observed area, as follows:

| Observation | Score (0) | Score (1) | Score (2) |
|---|---|---|---|
| Appearance | Blue, pale | Pink body, blue extremities | Pink all over |
| Pulse | Absent | Fewer than 100 bpm | Greater than 100 bpm |
| Grimace | No response | Some response | Cry, cough |
| Activity | Limp | Some flexion | Active motion |
| Respiration | Absent | Slow | Strong cry |

Following the one-minute evaluation, treatment is initiated, as necessary, according to the following scale:

| Apgar Score | Action |
|---|---|
| 8 to 10 | The majority of babies fall into this category. No medical attention is necessary, other than drying them and keeping them warm. |
| 5 to 7 | These babies need mild sensory stimulation and should receive oxygen to help them breathe. Most of these babies will improve as soon as they start breathing on their own. On rare occasions, further treatment may be necessary. |
| 3 to 4 | These babies need immediate ventilation with an oxygen mask. Their Apgar scores are monitored closely and further measures are taken as necessary. |
| 0 to 2 | These babies need immediate ventilation with an oxygen mask and continued ventilation through a breathing tube. Cardiac massage may be necessary, as well as an intravenous catheter for administering medications. |

*continued*

**Apgar Scores** *continued*

In the early 1950's, most expectant mothers having
cesarean deliveries received either spinal or general
anesthesia. In 1957, Dr. Apgar and her colleagues
determined that babies whose mothers received general
anesthesia during delivery scored lower than those
whose mothers received spinal anesthesia or epidural
anesthesia.

## Highly Fat-Soluble Narcotics

Sublimaze (fentanyl) and drugs in its related families sufentanil,
alfentanil, and remifentanil are fast acting pain relievers. They
have recently become popular in developed countries and are
used when epidural analgesia cannot be provided (for example,
when the mother's blood is not clotting properly) or when the
mother is too apprehensive about receiving the epidural needle
in her back. These drugs provide relief very quickly; their main
advantage is that the mother retains most of the drug in her body
and only a very small amount goes to the baby.

The disadvantages of fentanyl and its related drugs are that
they do not provide the same level of pain relief as an epidural,
and the pain relief they do provide does not last that long; therefore, they are typically administered intravenously as a continuous infusion or patient-controlled intravenous analgesia.

## Nubain (Nalbuphine)

Nubain (nalbuphine) is sometimes used for pain relief when
women attempt to deliver their babies naturally but ask for an

## Opioids Used for Labor Pain Relief

| Drug | Usual Dose Intravenous (IV) / Intramuscular (IM) | Onset (IV, IM) | Duration of Pain Relief | Comments |
|---|---|---|---|---|
| Morphine | 2–5 mg (IV) 10 mg (IM) | 3–5 min (IV) 20–40 min (IM) | 1–2 hours | May cause respiratory depression in the baby |
| Demerol (meperidine) | 25–50 mg (IV) 50–100 mg (IM) | 5–10 min (IV) 40–45 min (IM) | 2–4 hours | May cause depression in the baby if delivery occurs between 1 and 4 hours after administration |
| Sublimaze (fentanyl) | 25–50 mcg (IV) 100 mcg (IM) | 2–3 min (IV) 10 min (IM) | 30–60 minutes | 75 to 100 times more potent than morphine and 800 times more than Demerol; neonatal depression (if any) disappears quickly |

analgesia to help them get through the natural delivery. Although this drug can cause sleepiness in the mother, it is unlikely to cause depression in the baby.

### *Stadol (Butorphanol)*

Stadol (butorphanol) is similar to Nubain. It is a useful drug but, like Nubain, it causes extreme sleepiness in the mother.

## Tranquilizers

### Phenothiazines

Drugs in the phenothiazines family are occasionally used to eliminate the nausea and vomiting caused by Demerol.

### Valium and Versed (Benzodiazepines)

Sedatives in the benzodiazepine family, including Valium and Versed, have been used in conjunction with opioids for labor and delivery pain. These drugs help relax and calm expectant mothers. Valium remains in the baby's system for a long time (between 24 and 48 hours). Anesthesiologists have recently been using a short-acting drug in the same group, called Versed (midazolam), which only remains in the baby's system for six hours. The usual doses of Valium and Versed are 2–10 mg intravenously and 1–5 mg intravenously, respectively. At these doses, both drugs typically take effect within 5 minutes.

## Local Anesthetics

In addition to the drugs mentioned previously, there are five local anesthetic drugs that are used during labor and vaginal deliveries and cesarean births: bupivacaine, ropivacaine, levobupivacaine, lidocaine, and chloroprocaine. These drugs are used in the epidural, spinal, and combined spinal epidural techniques for labor, delivery, and cesarean section. They are also used to numb the perineum when an episiotomy is performed and also to repair the episiotomy incision.

These drugs are widely used because they do not cross the placenta in large amounts, and therefore have minimal effect on the babies. They are often given in combination with opioids.

## Other Medications

### Pitocin

Pitocin is often thought of as the drug used to induce labor. In addition to this purpose, Pitocin is also used to quicken the delivery of the placenta and contraction of the uterus after delivery of the baby.

# Labor and Delivery Analgesia and Anesthesia Techniques

Two types of analgesia and anesthesia techniques are used during labor and delivery: general and regional. General anesthesia is a technique in which gas and an intravenous sleeping drug are administered to expectant mothers so they are asleep during the delivery of their babies. Regional analgesia and anesthesia techniques such as the continuous spinal analgesia/anesthesia, epidural analgesia, and combined spinal epidural are techniques that enable expectant mothers to remain awake during the delivery of their babies. They provide pain relief by causing a loss of sensation in the lower region of the mother's body. Regional techniques are becoming more popular for labor and delivery for the following reasons:

- Mothers are looking for the ideal pain relief.

- With modern techniques, the amount of local anesthetic used for the epidural, the continuous spinal, and the combined spinal epidural techniques is extremely small and is mixed with narcotics. This gives the expectant mother effective pain relief with very little numbness. Mothers are able to push when the proper time comes. This can be described as "tailor-made pain relief," where anesthesiologists can select the technique and adjust the medication according to the expectant mother's needs.

- Minimal amounts of the drugs cross the placenta, resulting in few incidences of neonatal depression.

In this section, we'll explore the following types of analgesic and anesthetic techniques used during labor and delivery and their advantages and disadvantages:

- Continuous spinal analgesia/anesthesia

- Epidural analgesia

- Combined spinal epidural ("walking epidural")

- General anesthesia

At the end of this chapter we have included three illustrations. The first shows a cross section of the spine, illustrating the areas where spinal and epidural needles are inserted. The next

## What About Transcutaneous Nerve Stimulation (TENS)?

The Transcutaneous Nerve Stimulation (known as TENS) technique has been used for chronic pain relief, as well as relief of acute pain following surgery. With this technique, slight electrical impulses are applied to nerve endings through small wires taped to the skin. This technique has been tried as a pain reliever during labor and delivery, with varying degrees of success. Because of its inconsistent results, this technique has not become popular as an obstetric analgesia in the U.S.

two illustrations show correct body positioning of the expectant mother for effective epidural insertion.

The spinal and epidural techniques are described in the order in which they were introduced for use during deliveries.

## *Continuous Spinal Analgesia/Anesthesia*

As Dr. Koller was respected as the father of local anesthetics, James Leonard Corning was also respected as the father of the spinal anesthetic technique. Corning was born in Stamford, Connecticut in 1855, nine years after W. G. T. Morton demonstrated the use of ether in a general surgical case in Boston. Corning first demonstrated the use of cocaine as a spinal anesthetic in 1885, as a neurologist practicing in New York City. Although Corning was described as the father of spinal anesthesia, Dr. August Bier made the spinal anesthesia popular for surgeries. Dr. Bier administered spinal anesthesia with cocaine to his resident, and his resident returned the favor by administering the same on him. They discovered that this form of anesthesia was effective when they pulled on each other's pubic hair, pushed and pulled on the testes, and delivered sharp blows to the shins with a hammer. However, they both experienced horrible headaches and vomiting the next day, a condition we now call a post-spinal headache. (Today, we use a small needle tip—shaped like a pencil point—which greatly reduces the incidence of headache.)

Although cocaine was by now used extensively for general surgical patients, it was Dr. S. A. Cosgrove who first used spinal anesthesia for labor delivery. He discovered that because the anesthesia's effects were short-lived, he could use it only for the last part of the delivery; the expectant mother still felt pain during the first stage of labor. This technique became known as a "saddle block," named for the loss of feeling in the area that contacts the saddle when you are sitting on a horse.

The search continued for a technique by which a continuous spinal anesthesia could be used. Eventually, Dr. W. T. Lemmon from Philadelphia discovered a way to administer spinal anesthesia continuously: he threaded a tube through the spinal needle, through which a local anesthetic could be administered.

## *Advantages of Continuous Spinal Analgesia/Anesthesia*

The advantages of the continuous spinal analgesia/anesthesia technique in obstetrics are:

- The technique is reliable and easy to administer.

- It works very quickly, sometimes before the next contraction begins.

- The expectant mother remains awake, avoiding the problems associated with inserting breathing tubes in unconscious patients. (We will talk more about breathing tubes in the section "General Anesthesia.")

- Less drug is needed to achieve the same numbing effect as other techniques such as the epidural.

- Because a small amount of anesthetic is used, less is transferred to the baby.

## *Disadvantages of Continuous Spinal Analgesia /Anesthesia*

The disadvantages of the continuous spinal analgesia/anesthesia technique are:

- With prolonged use, the legs may become very numb, even if only a small amount of anesthetic is used.

- Because of the speed with which this technique works, some women become uneasy with the idea of being numb so quickly.

- Blood pressure drops quickly if a large amount of anesthetic is used. The rapid drop in blood pressure may
  cause nausea and vomiting. To prevent these uncomfortable side effects, your anesthesiologist will quickly treat
  your drop in blood pressure.

- Continuous spinal analgesia/anesthesia is associated with
  higher incidences of post-spinal headache; therefore, it is
  used in rare circumstances, such as the unlikely event of
  an accidental dural tap while performing the epidural
  analgesia technique.

## What is a Dural Tap?

The dura mater is a membrane that encases the spinal
cord and helps contain the spinal fluid. In the continuous spinal anesthesia/analgesia procedure, this membrane is intentionally punctured. In an epidural
analgesia procedure, the needle is inserted into the
"epidural space," the area just outside the dura; however, the epidural needle can accidentally puncture the
dural membrane.

An accidental or intentional puncture of the dura
mater is called a "dural tap." Both intended and unin-
tended dural taps can be associated with post-spinal
headache. (See illustration at end of chapter.)

### *Preparation for Continuous Spinal Analgesia/Anesthesia*

A typical epidural anesthetic tray used for this technique consists of washing equipment, a sterile drape, local anesthetics, gauze, an epidural needle, and an epidural catheter (tube) used to administer the anesthetics.

With this technique, the expectant mother's position is very important. Many anesthesiologists prefer the mother to be sitting for this procedure or lying on her side. If she sits, her legs should be over the side of the bed or delivery table and her feet on a stool. With help from the nurse, she will be asked to bend her back, bringing her chest toward her knees as much as possible; this position opens up the back for easy placement of the needle. (See illustrations at end of chapter.)

The anesthesiologist feels the mother's lower back to locate the best place to insert the epidural needle, then washes her back with a cold iodine solution or, if the mother is allergic to iodine, another antiseptic solution. As the solution dries, the anesthesiologist places a sterile plastic drape over the mother's back and prepares the drugs that will be used for the procedure.

A local anesthetic is injected through a tiny needle to numb the area, and feels like a bee sting. From then on, the mother feels no pain, only pressure as the epidural needle is inserted. When the anesthesiologist sees clear fluid coming through the epidural needle, he or she knows that the needle is in the right place. The anesthesiologist inserts an epidural catheter through the epidural needle, withdraws the epidural needle, and administers a small amount of local anesthetic and opioid narcotics through the catheter. Occasionally, it takes more than one attempt to complete this process because the spaces in the back are very narrow and the anesthesiologist has to ensure the needles are inserted in the proper place.

Anesthesiologists understand it is difficult to stay still during this period, particularly during contractions. However, it is very important to remain still during the entire process, especially when the needle is inserted, to ensure proper placement of the epidural needle and catheter.

If the mother was sitting, the anesthesiologist lets her lie down after the procedure is completed, checks her blood pressure and pulse, and looks for the ever-important "smiling sign" that means labor pain is subsiding. The nurse monitors the baby's heart rate. The mother is asked to lie on her side to prevent the uterus from pressing on the larger blood vessels and decreasing the flow of blood to the baby.

Because of the headaches associated with this technique, its intentional use is rare; this technique is more commonly used when the dura mater has accidentally been punctured during the epidural analgesia technique. In this case, the epidural catheter can be inserted into the spinal space through the epidural needle and used as a continuous spinal method of medication delivery instead.

Throughout labor and delivery, additional medication is administered through the catheter as necessary. The nurse continually monitors the mother's responses to the anesthesia, using devices that measure blood pressure, pulse, and fetal heart rate. The anesthesiologist stops administering medication through the catheter after the baby is delivered. If the mother still needs pain relief after the delivery, her obstetrician or midwife may recommend an oral pain-killing drug in the codeine or aspirin family or one of the intramuscular or intravenous pain-killing drugs we discussed earlier in this chapter.

## Epidural Analgesia

Sometimes described as the "Cadillac" of regional anesthetic techniques, the epidural analgesia technique was first used in general surgical cases in 1926. The American College of Obstetrics and Gynecology believes that "of the various pharmacological methods used for pain relief during labor and delivery, the lumbar epidural block is the most effective and least depressant, allowing for an alert, participating mother."

The main difference between this technique and the continuous spinal analgesia/anesthesia technique is that the epidural needle is not inserted as far into the spinal space, resulting in fewer headaches. This technique is considered a "blind" technique, which I will explain in a moment.

### Advantages of Epidural Analgesia

The advantages of the epidural analgesia technique are:

- The expectant mother remains awake.

- The onset of pain relief is slower, which helps avoid the alarm some women experience with the continuous spinal analgesia/anesthesia method when they feel that the lower part of their body is getting numb so quickly.

- There is a smaller chance of post-spinal headache, nausea, and vomiting than with the continuous spinal analgesia/anesthesia technique.

- Like the continuous spinal analgesia/anesthesia procedure, the catheter remains in the mother's back throughout labor. A small amount of local anesthetic and opioid mixture can be administered through the catheter as a continuous infusion or as often as necessary.

### Disadvantages of Epidural Analgesia

The disadvantages of the epidural analgesia technique are:

- The epidural analgesia is a more complex technique. Occasionally, a catheter may accidentally be inserted into a vein; in this case, the catheter is removed and a new catheter is inserted.

- Pain relief is slower than with the continuous spinal analgesia/anesthesia (about 15 minutes); this may be viewed as a disadvantage for mothers who want immediate pain relief.

- If the dura mater is accidentally punctured, there is a greater chance of the mother experiencing a post-spinal headache. If there is an accidental dural puncture, some anesthesiologists may thread the catheter through the hole in the dura mater and continue the procedure as a continuous spinal analgesic/anesthetic technique.

### Preparation for Epidural Analgesia

Many obstetricians prefer to wait to administer the epidural analgesia until the expectant mother's cervix is at least five centimeters dilated. At that point, the expectant mother is asked to sit on the edge of the table or lie on her side with her back bent, bringing her chest toward her knees as much as possible. Her back is then cleaned in the same manner as with the continuous spinal analgesia/anesthesia technique. As I mentioned, this is a blind technique; to find the proper location of the epidural space, anesthesiologists use a method called "loss of resistance." The expectant mother will feel a prick, followed by a burning sensation that lasts for a few seconds. A feeling of painless pressure follows this as the epidural needle is inserted. When the needle passes through the tough ligaments and there is no more resistance, we know we are in the proper location, the epidural space. We then insert a catheter and remove the needle. Through the catheter we administer small amounts of local anesthetic at a time, asking the mother to tell us if she feels different or if she feels any strange sensation. Once she is comfortable, we start an infusion of a mixture of local anesthetic and opioid.

As in the continuous spinal technique, the expectant mother

should try to remain still while the anesthesiologist places the epidural needle and catheter. The process of placing the epidural usually takes less than five minutes; after that, the expectant mother can relax.

Throughout labor and delivery, the nurse continually monitors the mother's responses to the anesthesia, using devices that measure blood pressure, pulse, and fetal heart rate. The anesthesiologist stops administering medication through the epidural catheter and removes the catheter after the baby is delivered. If the mother still needs pain relief after the delivery, her obstetrician or midwife may recommend an oral pain-killing drug in the codeine or aspirin family or one of the intramuscular or intravenous pain-killing drugs we discussed earlier in this chapter.

## Combined Spinal Epidural ("Walking Epidural")

The "walking epidural" combines the spinal and epidural techniques, enabling women to walk around the labor floor without feeling any pain. With this technique, the spinal part provides quick pain relief and the epidural part provides flexibility in the amount of anesthetic administered throughout labor, without the complete numbness of the continuous spinal analgesia/anesthesia technique.

"It's quiet," said Jacques Moritz, staff obstetrician on the labor floor at St. Luke's-Roosevelt Hospital Center in Manhattan when interviewed by Nancy Shute for an article in the U.S. News and World Report. "Not long ago," he continued, "you would walk the hall and hear people screaming." He attributed the quiet to the "walking epidural," which offers a safe, painless alternative to what can otherwise be a very painful experience.

A fellow anesthesiologist experienced first hand the benefits of this technique. She relates her personal experience as follows:

"With the birth of my second daughter, I arrived at the hospital early, fearing a more rapid labor and missing my window of opportunity to get an epidural analgesia since I was now a multipara (a woman with multiple pregnancies). I was four centimeters dilated. As I walked, bent over and moaning with the contractions, my male colleague hustled me into my room and got the OK to place my epidural catheter. Relief was very quick in onset; I had no weakness in my legs whatsoever. I did not feel the contractions at all. My husband and I set off for a visit down to the main operating room to say Hi to my colleagues and nurses. I pushed an intravenous pole, and walked normally. My friends were amazed to see me walking with a big smile on my face in a pink hospital gown with an intravenous and an epidural catheter in place. If that wasn't an advertisement of the remarkable "walking epidural," I don't know what is. I did not really look like I was in labor since I was walking around without a care in the world. We spent some time in the operating room and then returned to the labor floor to have our baby. I sort of felt like a cheater, having babies painlessly. I sometimes entertain the notion of delivering my third child without an epidural just to see what it feels like to have the labor and delivery pain without the epidural. Then I come to my senses and think to myself that all that pain and the maternal response to it can't be good for the baby, and why suffer when you can safely be made very comfortable for the birth?"

At Brigham and Women's Hospital, we currently deliver more than ten thousand babies a year. More and more expectant mothers are requesting the combined spinal epidural technique. Mothers like the freedom this form of pain relief provides; they can walk around, rest, read, or otherwise painlessly await the birth of their babies.

### Advantages of Combined Spinal Epidural

The advantages of the combined spinal epidural technique are:

- Pain relief is quick.

- Like the epidural analgesia technique, anesthesiologists have a great deal of flexibility in how much anesthesia to administer throughout the labor, which is useful in cesarean deliveries.

- Even when labor is prolonged (16–18 hours), very little of the anesthetic drug is transferred to the baby.

- If the expectant mother has severe pain in the early stages of labor and does not become comfortable after receiving an intravenous narcotic, we can administer a combined spinal epidural to take care of the pain.

• A combined spinal epidural can be administered late in labor, even if the mother is 8–10 centimeters dilated.

### Disadvantages of Combined Spinal Epidural

The disadvantages of the combined spinal epidural technique are:

• The spinal part of the procedure provides immediate pain relief, making it difficult to determine whether the epidural catheter is placed correctly. Because there is a slight chance of placing the catheter in the epidural vein or outside of the epidural space, the combined spinal epidural technique may not be appropriate for all women. For example, if the baby is in distress and the obstetrician decides to complete the delivery through an emergency cesarean section, the anesthesiologist will be forced to provide general anesthesia if the epidural catheter is found to be in the wrong place. If the expectant mother has a condition that prevents the anesthesiologist from easily inserting the breathing tube during the emergency cesarean section procedure, an epidural technique may be ideal.

• Mothers may experience a post-spinal headache, especially when the epidural needle during the epidural part of the procedure accidentally punctures the dura. If the headache persists after a few days or if the headache is severe, the new mother should have a blood patch. A blood patch will alleviate the headache by patching the hole made by the epidural needle and increasing the pressure of spinal fluid inside the brain.

### Preparation for Combined Spinal Epidural

Preparation for the combined spinal epidural is similar to that of the epidural technique. In this procedure, two needles are used: one that is placed in the epidural space and another long spinal needle that is inserted through the epidural needle to puncture the dura. After the spinal fluid appears through the spinal needle, a very small amount of medication (local anesthetic and narcotic) is injected. Following this, the spinal needle is withdrawn, an epidural catheter is inserted, and the epidural needle is removed. When the expectant mother is uncomfortable, a continuous infusion of local anesthetic and opioid can immediately be administered through the epidural catheter. In some institutions, the epidural mixture is started immediately after the combined spinal epidural technique is completed. As with the continuous spinal and epidural techniques, the mother must try not to move while the epidural and spinal needles are inserted.

Throughout labor and delivery, the nurse continually monitors the mother's responses to the anesthesia, using devices that measure blood pressure, pulse, and fetal heart rate. The anesthesiologist stops administering local anesthetic and opioid following the delivery of the baby. If the mother still needs pain relief after the delivery, her obstetrician or midwife may recommend an oral pain-killing drug in the codeine or aspirin family or one of the intramuscular or intravenous pain-killing drugs we discussed earlier in this chapter. Instead of a continuous epidural infusion, patient controlled epidural analgesia has also been used with success.

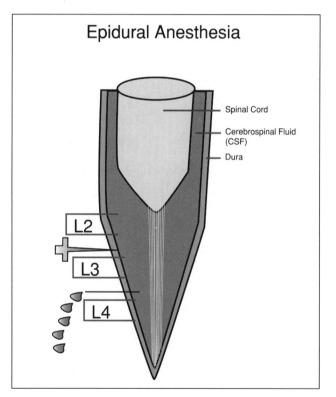

The spinal cord and its surrounding structure as it applies to regional anesthesia. The needle between L2 and L3 is the epidural needle. The needle between L3 and L4 is the spinal needle. The spinal cord normally ends above L2.

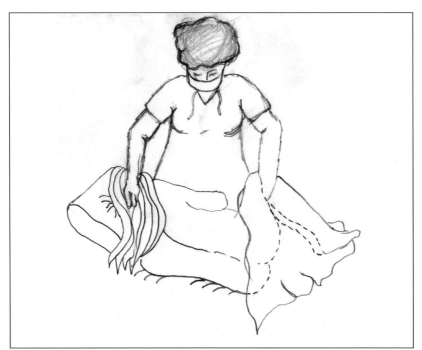

This illustration shows the mother's proper lying position for either epidural, spinal or combined spinal technique.

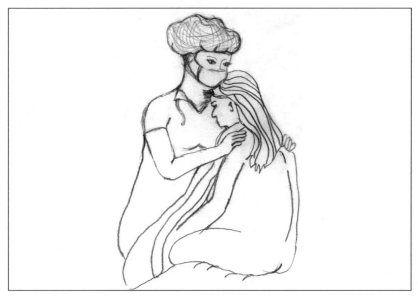

This illustration shows the mother's proper sitting position for either epidural, spinal or combined spinal technique.

# Spinal, Epidural, and Combined Spinal Epidural Techniques: A Comparison

| Continuous Spinal Anesthesia/Analgesia | Epidural Analgesia | Combined Spinal Epidural Anesthesia |
| --- | --- | --- |
| Simple and rapid | Complex; more difficult to ensure proper placement of epidural needle | Complex, but easier to ensure proper placement of epidural needle than with the epidural analgesia technique |
| Dural puncture is part of the procedure, resulting in greater incidences of headache | Dural puncture is avoided if possible, resulting in fewer incidences of headache | Dural puncture is made with a very small needle the shape of a pencil point; however, the combination of the spinal and epidural techniques results in fewer incidences of headache |
| Minimal amount of drug administered; therefore, less drug is absorbed by both the mother and the baby | Larger quantity of drug is administered, resulting in higher levels of the drug in both the mother and the baby, but still within safe limits | Minimal amount of drug is administered; therefore, less drug is absorbed by both the mother and the baby |
| Mother remains awake | Mother remains awake | Mother remains awake |
| Drop of blood pressure is common, resulting in nausea and vomiting; immediate treatment of drop in blood pressure is necessary | Drop of blood pressure is uncommon, resulting in few incidences of nausea and vomiting | Drop of blood pressure is uncommon, resulting in few incidences of nausea and vomiting |
| Quick onset | Slow onset | Quick onset |
| Immediate loss of sensory and motor power, which may be uncomfortable for some mothers | Sensory and motor loss are gradual | Sensory and motor loss are gradual and uncommon |

## General Anesthesia

General anesthesia, a combination of inhaled gas and intravenous sleeping drug, is sometimes administered during cesarean deliveries. There are two types of cesarean deliveries: elective and emergency. For elective cases, we can use any of the spinal, epidural, or combined spinal epidural techniques discussed earlier, as well as general anesthesia in certain circumstances. For emergency deliveries, we can use the continuous spinal or epidural techniques, or general anesthesia, depending upon the urgency of the situation.

### A Great Responsibility

An anesthesiologist's responsibility during a cesarean delivery is enormous. Not only is he or she looking after the welfare of the mother but also of the baby (sometimes multiple babies!). Planning the anesthesia technique to be used is a joint effort between the obstetrician, the anesthesiologist, and the expectant mother. The anesthesiologist should explain that local anesthetic procedures such as the spinal, epidural, and combined spinal epidural techniques are safer than general anesthesia; however, when circumstances require the use of general anesthesia, early planning by both physician and mother will help lower the risks.

### Fasting Before Surgery

During active labor it is better to have only ice chips or water, especially if general anesthesia is necessary. This recommendation to fast during labor or before surgery is one of the most controversial issues in the obstetric anesthesia practice. As mentioned earlier, pregnancy causes significant physiological changes, especially in the gastrointestinal system. Pregnancy delays gastric emptying in labor and increases gastric acidity. In one study, chunks of solid food were found during an ultrasound after 24 hours of fasting. This becomes significant if an expectant mother needs a breathing tube for an emergency cesarean delivery under general anesthetic—solid bits of food or liquid with a high acid content can enter the windpipe as the anesthesiologist is inserting the breathing tube. As long as the anesthesiologist is conservative, this will not happen frequently.

Members of the Society of Obstetric Anesthesia and Perinatology feel it is appropriate to avoid eating even a light meal or drinking milk for six or more hours before undergoing elective cesarean procedures.

So what can you eat? Expectant mothers may continue to have fruit juice, crackers and broth, or other lights foods, but should avoid heavy solids or foods with a high fat content when admitted for induction or observation to the labor and delivery unit. Once the mother has reached active labor (uterine contractions with cervical dilation) or has had an epidural catheter placed, obstetricians usually advise her to limit her intake to water or ice chips.

High-risk patients (for example, obese women or expectant mothers who need general anesthesia) should not have any solid food after they are admitted on the labor floor. This policy is primarily meant to serve as a guide for practitioners on the labor and delivery unit. As approved by the Obstetric Care Committee at Brigham and Women's Hospital in 1992, the obstetrician and anesthesiologist may alter this guideline as necessary to the individual needs of each expectant mother.

### *Advantages of General Anesthesia*

The advantages of general anesthesia are:

- It is quick and reliable.

- It is more easily controlled.

- There is little chance of a drop in blood pressure.

### *Disadvantages of General Anesthesia*

The disadvantages of general anesthesia are:

- The expectant mother and her partner cannot be involved in the birthing process.

- Because the expectant mother is unconscious, there is a small chance that she may breathe solid, semi-solid, or acid contents through the trachea and ultimately into her lungs.

- It may be difficult to insert the breathing tube.

- Anesthesiologists administer a minimal amount of anesthetic to avoid depression of the baby; however, if the delivery takes longer than expected, there is a chance the baby may become depressed and may need to be resuscitated.

- Mothers may experience nausea and vomiting after they regain consciousness.

## *Preparation for General Anesthesia*

The anesthesiologist first puts a mask over the expectant mother's face and asks her to take deep breaths of oxygen, then administers an intravenous drug to put her to sleep. Just before the expectant mother falls asleep, the assistant applies some pressure with his or her fingers just below the mother's Adam's apple to help prevent the mother from inhaling any stomach contents into her lungs as the anesthesiologist inserts the breathing tube. During surgery, the anesthesiologist continually monitors her blood pressure, heart rate, oxygen saturation, and carbon dioxide saturation; when surgery is complete, the anesthesiologist turns off the flow of anesthetic and brings the mother back to consciousness. She may be a bit groggier following the general anesthesia than when other types of anesthesia are administered.

# Do Other Anesthesia Options Exist for Cesarean Deliveries?

A one-shot spinal anesthesia is becoming popular for elective cesarean section deliveries. With this technique, the expectant mother's back is prepared the same way as in the continuous spinal, epidural, and combined spinal epidural techniques. A small amount of local anesthetic is administered through a needle in the back. A small pencil point needle is introduced to puncture the dura. After the cerebrospinal fluid appears, a small amount of local anesthetic and opioid mixture is injected. No catheter is used in this technique.

The advantages of the one-shot spinal anesthesia are that this technique is easy to administer, is fast acting and reliable, transfers very little medication to the baby, and, because the mother remains awake, there is little chance of her inhaling any stomach contents.

The disadvantages of this technique are a significant drop in the mother's blood pressure, nausea and vomiting, and a small chance of headache. Immediate treatment of the drop in blood pressure is important. Also, because no catheter is used, this technique is not as flexible as the continuous spinal, epidural, or combined spinal epidural techniques in the amount of drug that can be administered.

The continuous spinal, epidural, or combined spinal epidural techniques can still be used for cesarean deliveries. These techniques are the same as for vaginal deliveries; however, for cesarean deliveries, a larger dose of local anesthetic mixed with opioid is used. This larger dose extends the numbness up to the chest. With any of these techniques, the expectant mother may experience a tugging sensation as the obstetrician removes the baby from her uterus, but should feel no pain. Just before the baby is delivered, the expectant mother will feel pressure under her rib cage as the obstetrician presses on her upper abdomen to push the baby through the incision. She may then experience nausea or discomfort as the obstetrician moves the uterus around to repair the incision.

## *Post-operative Pain Relief*

Post-operative pain relief following a cesarean delivery has changed dramatically in many hospitals. Pain-killing medications are typically given through the spinal needle or the epidural catheter. This avoids the drowsiness caused by other types of pain relievers, is effective for 12–18 hours, and enables the new mother to get out of bed and start interacting with her baby. Following the initial dose of pain medication, mothers can take additional pain relievers by mouth; these pain relievers are usually enough to keep the mother comfortable for the rest of her hospital stay.

# Closing Words

I have always believed that it is the expectant mother who makes the ultimate decision regarding the pain relief for her labor and delivery. I hope that this book has given you the knowledge you need to choose a pain relief method that is right for you, answered some questions you may have had along the way, and helped you feel more comfortable about the medical procedures behind this wonderful event. Remember, your obstetrician, your midwife, and your anesthesiologist are there to help.

I pray and wish for all the best for you and your new baby.

# Questions and Answers

Q.   How do I decide which labor and delivery pain relief option to choose?

A.   Consult with the obstetrician and/or midwife you will be seeing throughout your pregnancy, talk to your friends and colleagues, and contact an anesthesiologist at your hospital. Attend childbirth education classes and read the literature provided by your hospital. If you want to try natural childbirth, your anesthesiologist may still want to see you to ask a few questions.

Q.   I am planning for natural childbirth; will you be able to help me if I fail?

A.   First of all, if you begin the labor and delivery process using a natural childbirth method but during labor you feel that this

**69**

method is not adequate for your pain relief, please do not think you have failed. If you change your mind during labor, an anesthesiologist would be happy to help you, provided your labor is not so advanced that delivery is imminent.

Q.   What is cervical incompetence?

A.   Cervical incompetence is a condition in which the expectant mother's cervix has either dilated prematurely, or is too thin (effaced). In either case, a procedure called cervical cerclage is done to prevent pre-term labor and midterm miscarriages. This procedure involves stitching (suturing) the cervix, and is usually done when expectant mothers are 12–14 weeks pregnant. Both regional and general anesthesia can be used for this procedure. At Brigham and Women's Hospital, spinal anesthesia is the preferred method for this surgery. The women are conscious, thereby greatly diminishing the likelihood of nausea, vomiting, and aspiration of stomach content.

In routine cases, the sutures are removed 37–38 weeks into the pregnancy, usually with no need for anesthesia. However, in rare cases, analgesics and tranquilizers may be necessary. Occasionally, spinal or general anesthesia is used.

Q.   What can I eat or drink during labor?

A.   During labor, and especially if you receive pain relief medication, your stomach and digestive tract empty themselves of solid food and liquid much slower than normal. To prevent aspiration, your obstetrician may only allow you to consume ice chips and water during active labor, especially if there is a chance that you will undergo general anesthesia for a cesarean delivery.

Q. When can I have my epidural?

A. This is one of the most common questions asked of anesthesiologists by expectant mothers, and is also one of the most controversial. Obstetricians and midwives vary considerably on their views of when to administer pain relief by regional analgesia techniques. In my hospital, some obstetricians will let the expectant mother have pain relief in the early stage of cervical dilation if the mother is extremely uncomfortable, whereas other obstetricians wait until the expectant mother's cervix is more dilated. Studies have shown that the use of low concentrations of local anesthetics and narcotics did not effect the uterine contractions. If you are really uncomfortable after the use of intravenous pain medication, you should ask your obstetrician or midwife about the possibility of getting pain relief from the anesthesiologist.

Q. I thought I could have the epidural for pain relief, but my anesthesiologist says I should not. What is my alternative?

A. If you have any systemic disease, such as blood clotting problems, back problems, or neurological problems, you must consult with an anesthesiologist. In some rare circumstances, the continuous spinal, epidural, or combined spinal epidural techniques should not be used. In those circumstances, the anesthesiologist will provide intravenous analgesia during the first stage of labor; then, during the second stage, the obstetrician might be able to help you with different blocks. For some cesarean deliveries, general anesthesia may be the only option. With other systemic diseases, like diabetes, cardiac disease, or respiratory disease, regional analgesia may be a better option. Anesthesiologists choose anesthesia and analgesia methods based on each mother's individual situation; that is why it is so important to provide an accurate medical history during your first consultation with your obstetrician.

Q.  What are the incidences of accidental dural puncture headache? What will happen if I get a headache?

A.  Incidences of accidental dural tap vary among different hospitals. In our hospital, the incidences are 0.5-1%. If an accidental dural puncture happens, we typically insert an epidural catheter through the hole made by the epidural needle and then remove the needle. We use a very small amount of local anesthetic and narcotics until the delivery of the baby, and keep the catheter in place for a certain length of time afterward to assist in the healing of the dura. This provides an excellent analgesia with very little leg weakness and reduces the incidences of post-dural puncture headache and the need for a blood patch.

If the mother gets a headache after delivery, we first have her drink plenty of caffeinated fluids and give her pain medication for the headache. If she does not feel relief, we do an epidural blood patch by placing an epidural needle, removing a small amount of blood from the mother's arm, injecting the blood through the epidural needle, and removing the epidural needle. Although the success rate is high, in some cases a second blood patch may be necessary.

Q.   How much will it hurt to have an epidural?

A.   The epidural should not hurt much. Before we insert the epidural needle (which is large), we numb the skin and the deeper layer using a local anesthetic so that the epidural needle placement does not hurt. We try to make this procedure as comfortable as possible; please tell the anesthesiologist if you feel pain during the procedure.

Q.   How will you know if the catheter has reached a vein? What will happen to me?

A.   If the catheter is in a blood vessel, the blood will appear in the catheter. However, if we are not absolutely sure, we administer a test dose of anesthetic; if the catheter is in a blood vessel, your heart will beat faster and you might feel strange sensations in your lips, tongue, and ears.

Q.   Will I have any back pain following the continuous spinal, epidural, or combined spinal epidural techniques?

A.    Two types of back pain are associated with any of these tech-
      niques: a localized back pain from the needle and a generalized
      back pain in the lower back. You may experience localized back
      pain following the use of the continuous spinal, epidural, or
      combined spinal epidural techniques, but this pain will disap-
      pear shortly after delivery. You may also experience generalized
      back pain. However, this pain is not necessarily attributed to
      the epidural; studies have shown that mothers who have natu-
      ral childbirth deliveries are as likely to experience generalized
      back pain as those who have epidurals. It seems that pregnancy
      itself can increase the incidences of back pain because softer
      ligaments contribute to back strain.

Q.    How will general anesthesia affect the baby?

A.    In the United States, general anesthesia is used only in rare
      cases like emergency cesarean deliveries or in situations where
      regional anesthesia cannot be used. When general anesthesia
      is administered, incidences of depression in the baby are
      unlikely, for two reasons: we typically use a light anesthesia and
      the time interval between the induction of anesthesia and deliv-
      ery of the baby is usually short. If a baby does have trouble,
      either the neonatologist or the anesthesiologist will be there to
      assist the baby.

Q.    What is a walking epidural? Do you use it in your hospital?

A.    The walking epidural is also called the combined spinal
      epidural and is covered in detail in this book. It is a technique

where a small amount of local anesthetic is mixed with a narcotic and administered using the combined spinal epidural
method. After these drugs are administered, the anesthesiologist performs tests to make sure the expectant mothers can
walk. Fetal heart rate is checked either from a remote control
method or by nurses every half an hour. In a few hospitals, the
walking epidural is done routinely. The greatest benefit of this
technique is that the mother experiences less numbness than
with the continuous spinal or epidural techniques. Yes, we do
perform this technique in our hospital.

Q.  Are all the pain relief techniques we discussed in this book
available at all hospitals?

A.  The pain relief techniques we discussed in this book should be
available wherever anesthesiologists practice.

# Resources and Recommended Book Reading

Lamaze International
2025 M Street NW, Suite 800
Washington, DC 20036-3309
800-368-4404
www.lamaze.org

## Web Sites

birthworks.org

childbirth.org

icea.org

mayohealth.org

women.com

# Books (listed alphabetically)

*The Birth Partner: Everything You Need to Know to Help a Woman Through Childbirth* by Penny Simkin

*Birthing from Within: An Extra-Ordinary Guide to Childbirth Preparation* by Pam England

*The Complete Book of Pregnancy and Childbirth* by Sheila Kitzinger

*Gentle Birth Choices: A Guide to Making Informed Decisions About Birthing Centers, Birth Attendants, Water Birth, Home Birth, Hospital Birth* by Barbara Harper

*A Good Birth, A Safe Birth: Choosing and Having the Childbirth Experience You Want* by Diana Korte

*Pregnancy Childbirth and the Newborn: The Complete Guide* by Penny Simkin

*What to Expect When You're Expecting* by Arlene Eisenberg

# Glossary

**Abdominal delivery**—*See* cesarean delivery.

**Amniotic membrane**—The membrane that covers the amniotic sac containing the baby and the amniotic fluid.

**Anesthesia and analgesia**—These terms are different in relation to the intensity of sensory and motor block. Anesthesia is used when a more complete pain block is essential, as in cesarean sections; in this situation, more local anesthetic is administered than in a vaginal delivery. Analgesia is used when less pain block can be tolerated, as in labor and vaginal deliveries; in this situation, only enough local anesthetic is given to control labor and delivery pain without completely numbing the area.

**Apgar score**—A method by which the appearance, pulse, facial expression, activity level, and respiration of a baby are assessed one minute and five minutes after birth. The baby is assigned a score and treatment is initiated as necessary according to the assigned score.

**Aspiration**—The breathing of stomach contents into the lungs.

**Blood patch**—The patching of the dural hole made by the epidural needle or, more rarely, the spinal needle. A blood patch is only used if there is a post-dural puncture headache.

**Catheter**—See epidural catheter.

**Cervical dilation**—The dilation of the cervix. When the expectant mother is in active labor, the cervix should dilate one centimeter per hour. She is considered fully dilated when her cervix is 10 centimeters dilated.

**Cervical cerclage**—See cervical incompetence.

**Cervical incompetence**—A condition in which the cervical muscles have dilated prematurely, or are not strong enough to hold the baby in the uterus throughout the pregnancy. To prevent pre-term labor or miscarriage, the obstetrician will stitch (suture) the cervix closed when expectant mothers are 12–14 weeks pregnant. This procedure is called a cervical cerclage.

**Cesarean delivery**—A procedure in which the baby is delivered abdominally through an incision in the uterine wall. This is also referred to as abdominal delivery.

**Coagulation**—Clot formation of the blood. To prepare for blood loss during delivery, blood coagulates more readily during pregnancy.

**Collagen**—A gelatinous material found in connective tissue, cartilage, and bone.

**Combined spinal epidural**—A regional anesthesia technique that combines the benefits of the continuous spinal analgesia/anesthesia technique (quick, effective pain relief and lesser amounts of medication) with the benefits of the epidural analgesia technique (lower incidence of headache). This technique allows the expectant mother to walk around during labor, and is becoming more popular in many hospitals.

**Continuous intravenous infusion**—A technique in which a fixed amount of local anesthetic and opioid is given to the expectant mother intravenously for labor and delivery pain relief.

**Continuous spinal analgesia/anesthesia**—The first regional anesthesia technique to be used for labor and delivery pain relief. In this technique, an epidural needle punctures the dura mater. When spinal fluid becomes visible, a catheter is introduced, and small amounts of local anesthetic and opioid narcotics are administered through the catheter. This technique provides quick pain relief but is associated with high incidences of post-spinal headache.

**Dura mater**—The outermost layer that covers the spinal cord and spinal fluid.

**Dural tap**—Puncture of the dura mater either by epidural needle or spinal needle. Intentional and accidental dural taps are associated with post-spinal headache.

**Epidural analgesia**—A regional analgesia technique that was developed after the continuous spinal analgesia/anesthesia technique. Unlike the continuous spinal technique, the dura mater is not intentionally punctured in the epidural, resulting in fewer post-spinal headaches. This technique provides slower pain relief than the continuous spinal analgesia/anesthesia technique, but because less drug is administered, less is transferred to the baby.

**Epidural catheter**—In obstetric regional anesthesia and analgesia, a tube that is inserted through an epidural needle into the expectant mother's back. This tube is used to administer local anesthetic and opioid mixtures to provide pain relief during labor and delivery.

**Epidural space**—The space outside the dural membrane.

**Episiotomy**—A procedure in which an incision is made in the perineum just before the baby is delivered. This procedure is performed to prevent tearing of the vagina and the vaginal wall; the episiotomy incision is easier to repair than a vaginal tear. A local anesthetic is injected directly into the region just before the incision is made to prevent pain during the incision and during the repair after delivery (if no regional anesthetics are used).

**Esophagus**—The tube beginning at the neck and extending to the stomach that carries food to the stomach. *See also* trachea.

**Ether anesthesia**—The oldest anesthetic vapor ever used for general surgical operations, labor and vaginal delivery and cesarean deliveries.

**Fellowship**—Specialized training in which a trained anesthesiologist completes one more year of residency (his or her fourth year of residency) in a particular subspecialty. In an obstetric anesthesia fellowship, trained residents spend this year in the obstetric unit.

**General anesthesia**—A technique where gas and an intravenous sleeping drug are administered to expectant mothers so they are asleep during the delivery of their babies. General anesthesia is no longer widely used in modern countries during childbirth and is reserved only for special circumstances, such as emergency cesarean deliveries.

**Induction**—The administration of local or general anesthetic during regional anesthesia, regional analgesia, or general anesthesia.

**Lamaze method**—A formalized method that uses relaxation, focus, breathing, and massage techniques to ease pain during labor and delivery. The techniques taught in this method can be used during natural childbirth and also during childbirth that is assisted by pain relief medications or anesthesia.

**Local anesthesia**—Anesthesia injected into a small, specific area of the body to numb only that area.

**Neonatal depression**—After the baby is delivered either vaginally or through a cesarean section, it is referred to as a neonate. Neonatal depression is a condition where the baby's physical, motor, and respiratory responses are below normal. These responses are measured using the Apgar scoring method one minute and five minutes after birth. See also Apgar score.

**Neonatologist**—A specialist who takes care of the neonates (babies that have just been delivered). These physicians have to complete a pediatric residency followed by a fellowship.

**Obstetric anesthesia**—Anesthesia or analgesia related to obstetrics.

**Opioid**—A pain-killing drug originally derived from the opium plant and now available in synthetic form.

**Patient-controlled intravenous analgesia**—A technique in which medications are administered intravenously. The patient controls the amount of medication that is administered by pushing a button attached to the intravenous tube. Patients that control their own medication flow tend to administer less of the drug than if they received a continuous infusion administered by a physician or nurse.

**Perineum**—The part of the body situated between the thighs at the outlet of the pelvis. The perineum is a triangular structure made of ligaments, tissue, and muscles supporting the vagina and rectum.

**Plasma**—A component of blood without red blood cells.

**Postpartum**—A stage that begins after the birth of the baby and the placenta. This is an important stage because most of the physiological changes that occur during pregnancy revert to a woman's pre-pregnant state a few days to a few weeks after delivery of her baby.

**Progesterone**—A female hormone that is present in the blood in small amounts, which increases dramatically during pregnancy and drops significantly before the labor starts.

**Psychoprophylaxis**—The preparation of the mind to deal with pain naturally. This term originated from the idea that if expectant mothers are properly educated about the labor and delivery process, stay relaxed and focused during labor and delivery, and have a good support system, they can cope with labor and delivery pain. Psychoprophylaxis was embraced by Fernand Lamaze and developed into the Lamaze technique that is taught today in many hospitals and birthing centers. See also Lamaze method.

**Regional anesthesia**—A local anesthetic is injected near a group of nerves to numb a larger area of the body more intensely.

**Spinal anesthesia**—*See* continuous spinal analgesia/anesthesia.

**Spinal space**—The innermost space containing the spinal cord and spinal fluid. The outermost space is the epidural space.

**Trachea**—The tube beginning at the neck and extending to the lungs that enables a person to breathe. See also esophagus.

**Twilight Sleep**—A technique in which a combination of morphine and scopolamine was used to induce a semi-conscious state. Morphine provided a certain amount of pain relief, whereas scopolamine was associated with amnesia so that if the patient did experience any pain, he or she did not remember it.

**Vaginal delivery**—The vagina is a part of the birth canal that extends from the uterus to the vulva. Delivery via the birth canal is called vaginal delivery.

**Walking Epidural**—*See* combined spinal epidural.

# Bibliography

*American Society of Anesthesiologist Newsletter* 1997;61(9).

Apgar, Virginia et al. Comparison of regional and general anesthesia in obstetrics. *Journal of the American Medical Association* 1957, 2155.

Borst, C. *Catching Babies: The Professionalization of Childbirth 1870-1920.* Cambridge, Massachusetts, 1995.

Dick-Read, Grantly. *Childbirth Without Fear.* New York, 1944.

Freedman L.Z., Ferguson V.M. The question of painless childbirth in primitive cultures. Yale Medical School, 1949.

Fülöp-Miller R. (translated by Paul C. & Paul E.). *Triumph Over Pain.* New York, 1938.

Harper, Barbara. *Gentle Birth Choices.* Vermont: Healing Arts Press Inc., 1994.

Karmel, Marjorie. *Thank You, Dr. Lamaze.* New York, 1976.

Lamaze, Fernand. *Painless Childbirth: The Lamaze Method*. New York, 1970.

Leavitt, J.W. *Brought to Bed: Childbearing in America 1750 to 1950*. New York, 1986.

Lindstrom, C. and Moore, D.C. Trends in obstetrical anesthesia following the acceptance of a twenty-four hour physician anesthesia service. *Obstetric and Gynecology 1957*. March-April:63.

Lyman, H.M. *Artificial Anaesthesia*. New York, 1881.

Melzack, Ronald et al. Labour is still painful after prepared childbirth training. *Canadian Medical Association Journal*. 1981; 125:357.

Melzack, Ronald et al. Severity of labour pain: influence of physical as well as psychologic variables. *Canadian Medical Association Journal*. 1984;130:579.

Pope Pius XII. Three religious and moral questions about anesthesia. Tipo grafia Poliglotta. Vatican, Rome, 1958.

Sandelowski, M. *Pain, Pleasure and American Childbirth: From the Twilight Sleep to the Read Method, 1914-1960*. London, 1984.

Vandam, LD. On the origins of intrathecal anesthesia. *Regional Anesthesia and Pain Medicine*. 1998;23(4):335.

Wertz, D.C. and Wertz, R.W. *Lying-In: A History of Childbirth in America*. London, 1977.

# Index